Stay Naturally Healthy wi

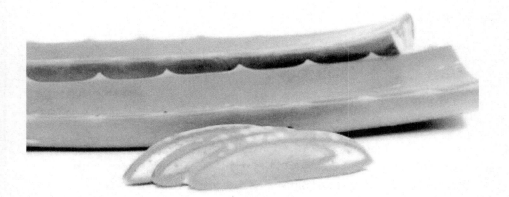

Dueep Jyot Singh

Healthy Learning Series

Mendon Cottage Books

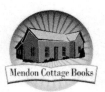

JD-Biz Publishing

Our books are available at

1. Amazon.com
2. Barnes and Noble
3. Itunes
4. Kobo
5. Smashwords
6. Google Play Books

Download Free Books!

http://MendonCottageBooks.com

Table of Contents

Introduction

A number of my friends asked me how Aloe Vera, which has long been in use in cosmetics, was never ever used in medicine, in modern times and in ancient times. I was astonished to hear that they did not know that Aloe Vera, which I considered all these years to be a very common useful healing herb, available right at hand was an excellent, important, and ready beneficial herb. But then familiarity breeds contempt.

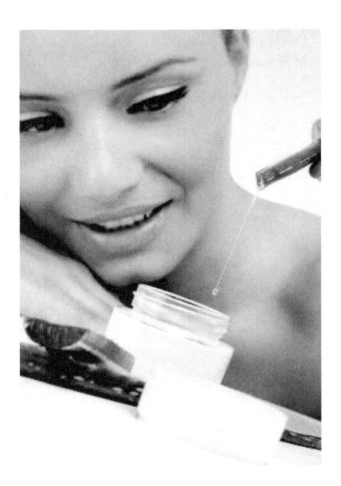

So this book is for all of them, to tell them all about the magic power of Aloe Vera, and how the gel, juice, and the concentrate has been in use for millenniums in order to cure diseases as well as prevent them.

And yes, in ancient times, especially in Greek, Roman, Egyptian, Indian, Chinese, Japanese, and Eastern as well as Western medicine, Aloe Vera was an integral part of the natural herb pantheon. The Egyptians and the Greeks called it the *cure all*. They used it for everything from curing sunburn to steadying their high blood pressure and it is a sad thing that science-based medicine is preventing the use of Aloe Vera to cure a number of chronic diseases and ordinary diseases naturally.

In Vietnam, you can recognize aloe under the name of Loe Hoi. In Greece, everybody knew about the healing powers of Aloe Vera in the times of Alexander when his teacher Aristotle told him to capture the island of Socotra where there was a native species of superior Aloe Vera growing. And this was around 2400 BC. Even at that time they knew all about the value of Aloe Vera gel, Aloe Vera juice, and took plenty of advantage of such rich sources of Aloe Vera growing wild, and being cultivated by the natives.

In ancient times, in many parts of the East, Aloe Vera was chopped up into small pieces, and fried in clarified butter. It was then given to the patients to relieve them of pain and cure them of a large number of diseases. It was also a secret weapon for all those beauties who wanted to stay eternally young.

This was done by eating a couple of pieces of Aloe Vera, fresh off the leaf, first thing in the morning. Many people who are going to taste Aloe Vera for the first time make faces because according to them, it is really bitter and eating Aloe Vera is an acquired taste. Well, the answer is you do not have to eat bitter Aloe Vera. Just keep watering your Aloe Vera plant, and the more you water it, the sweeter the inner gel is going to be. The water content diluted the bitter quality of the gel.

You can also add orange juice, lemon juice, or pineapple juice to aloe juice, when you are drinking it on an empty stomach, first thing in the morning. I added a little bit of rock candy to it, and that improves the taste.

The Aloe Vera products that you find on your supermarket shelves are definitely not the original stuff because they have preservatives as well as sweet smelling ingredients added to them.

Difference Between Aloe Vera Juice And Aloe Vera Gel

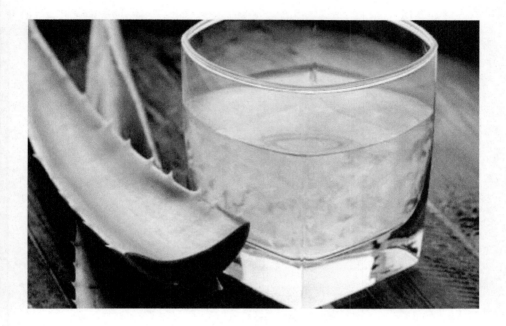

There is a difference between Aloe Vera juice and Aloe Vera gel. Aloe Vera gel is sticky, transparent, and viscous in nature. One could almost call it the pulp present between the upper and the lower portions of the leaf. Aloe Vera juice is present right under the outer covering of the leaf. You can scoop out the gel, with the help of a spoon, and scrape off the juice with the help of the same spoon. Both of these natural products are amazingly effective in helping you keep healthy.

The quantity of Aloe Vera juice that a healthy person can take starts with one teaspoonful in a day. After some time, you can increase the intake to three – four teaspoonfuls per day. Here is another way in which you can make pure Aloe Vera juice.

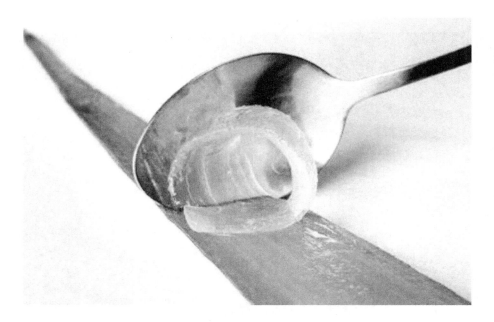

Aloe Vera Juice

Take fresh aloe gel from the leaves. Chop it up into small pieces, and mix it with a little bit of water. Whether you want thick juice or thin juice is going to depend on the amount of the water that you put in the gel. It takes anywhere between two – three months of a regular intake of this juice to start showing excellent and visible effects upon your body. That is because nature takes about this much time to help heal your body of any sort of infection, purify your blood, open up the pores of your skin, strengthen your immune system and it also helps in the regulation of your weight.

Also, if you suffer from chronic insomnia, here is a suggestion. Just add a teaspoonful of Aloe Vera juice to your daily diet. You may find yourself dropping off to sleep, but do not be surprised at the lower amount and hours of the sleep that you need. Even so, when you wake up in the morning, you are going to find yourself refreshed, energetic, and ready to take on a new day.

Aloe Vera was considered very precious in ancient times, because it was thought to cure any sort of disease and illness, permanently. The ancients claimed that this was so. Twenty first century medical science and modern-day doctors do not want to accept this fact; because that means that their chemical-based medicines will not be bought by their patients, if the diseases are healed permanently. And that is the reason why, people who start using natural remedies for the first time and do not know the proper dosage find themselves suffering from stomach upsets. And so they go to the hospital, where there is a doctor there to tell them *I told you so*. And then they think to themselves, of course, he is right, and alternative medicine is junk and bunk.

It is almost as bad as swallowing a bottle of antibiotics, when the dosage was half a tablet per day.

So anybody who tells you to drink a glass full of Aloe Vera juice could not care less about your health. That is because whether you are a child or an adult, you do not drink more than one spoonful at a time. You can add this to your glass of orange, lemon, squash, or any other juice.

This is normally taken on an empty stomach, first thing in the morning. And after you have done that, you are going to drink warm water, an hour after you have drunk this juice. This warm water is to support the assimilation of the Aloe Vera in your system. And now you can have your breakfast.

In the evening, if you want to take the juice, you are going to have it one hour after your dinner. And then after an hour, you are going to take a glass full of lukewarm water.

A word of caution here – as in any natural remedy, it is possible that you may find yourself suffering from a mild side effect. Most of us are so frightened with the onset of a possible stomach upset, or fever, or anything else, that we immediately stop the natural remedy because we dare not take a chance. Remember that this natural reaction is the body's way of telling you – all right then, you have given my weak and infected system some support from some natural healing product. The body is not used to it.

So there is going to be a normal reaction in the bio–physiological makeup of your body. Until the reaction takes place, the body is not going to throw off the results of the infection and begin the curing process.

The reaction is going to depend on the seriousness of the disease and the amount of infectious material present in the body, which has to be destroyed and removed from the body.

All these toxins are removed naturally by the body through excretion. The moment all these toxins are removed, your body is going to start feeling healthy and full of well-being. Again, this toxin removal is going to depend on how healthy your body was in the first place, and how severe the infection is.

Aloe Vera is capable of preventing infections as well as healing chronic diseases. But naturally, you need to be patient. And also, anybody who is under the impression that drinking huge quantities of Aloe Vera is going to heal them sooner, especially of chronic diseases, I am sorry but nature does not work that way. On the other hand, she is going to react even more, because you have poisoned your system with support medicines, which instead of being healers have now taken on the shape of inhibiting poisons.

I accompanied a friend of mine to the market, because she wanted a huge one liter bottle of Aloe Vera juice, to drink. When I told her that that was not done, she told me that doctors knew best. Please take my advice, because I have your best interests at heart. I am not selling you expensive medicines. I do not want you coming to my hospital, with the side effects of the drugs, for ailments which could have been cured with a regular small dose of Aloe Vera.

So, S. picked up a huge bottle of Aloe Vera juice and Aloe Vera gel. And then she smiled, because the brand Pharma company, which was selling this to her called it stabilized Aloe Vera gel.

According to them, they heated the product, had some preservatives added to it, and made sure that it kept for years and years. My friend, you need to forget all this marketing hype. You need to preserve the Aloe Vera gel, naturally. You need to stabilize it, after you have removed the gel from inside the leaf. This process has to be done within an hour of the removal of the gel because the more it is exposed to the open air, the less it is effective.

Put the gel in a glass bottle. Add a little bit of almond oil to it. You can also add wheat germ oil, if you want, as an alternative to almond oil. There you are, you have properly stabilized your gel, and the almond oil is going to preserve it, for years. Easy, is not it.

Even today, all over the East, you are going to find places where children were given one teaspoonful of Aloe Vera juice, diluted in a glass full of water since childhood, until they were 18 years of age. The idea was that they would keep healthy throughout their childhood, and as they reached their teens, with its accompanying hormonal changes, they would not suffer from any sort of teenage related ailments.

I tasted it for the first time when I was seven years old, because my grandmother had made traditional Aloe Vera pickles, sun-dried and good for one's health. She wanted my younger brother and me to have one piece, without fail, every day, so that we would keep healthy and hearty. We took one bite, and decided that this pickle was definitely not our cup of tea. So my grandmother threatened us that when we turned 13, and pimples began to make an appearance on our skin, we would then say – grandma was right!

By the way pimples never made an appearance on our skin, because we were not genetically prone to them, but even so a bit of Aloe Vera every day would not have harmed our skin, especially as we grew older!

This is the reason why Aloe Vera is such an integral part of the cosmetic industry today.

It was in 2004, when some agricultural Pioneer decided that Aloe Vera should be planted all over the desert area so that apart from a future financial profitable crop, it could be used to make healing medicines for the villagers of the villages, where medical aid was not readily available. Today, more than 170 villages in that particular desert area earn their livelihood through Aloe Vera, which is stabilized with the help of almond oil and send abroad, packed into expensive bottles, and then sent back to us to buy at hugely inflated rates! That is business!

It takes about two years for a plant to grow well enough to give you a good yield. One hectare can produce 10 – 12 tons of Aloe Vera leaves. But as I am not, and you are not starting up an Aloe Vera plantation, we can plant a plant or two or three, right in our gardens, in some containers or in some pots, for domestic consumption.

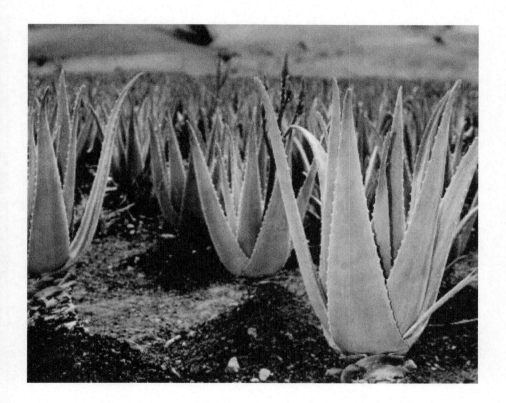

The best thing about Aloe Vera is that it does not need lots of water at all. So as half of the plants in my garden are succulents, I can go off on trips, occasionally, for a couple of days, without fearing that when I come back, my garden is going to be filled up with dead and dying plants.

And when I have to harvest some gel from one particular well growing plant, I begin watering it in the morning, in the afternoon, and at night, about a week before harvesting, so that the gel is sweet. The next Sunday, armed with a sharp knife, and gloves, the leaves are going to be harvested, the knife used to remove the top epidermis, the gel scooped out in a glass bottle, two tablespoons full of wheat germ oil added to it, and the bottle labeled with the date and time. That is that! A whole month's supply of aloe Vera collected in a couple of hours.

Why is the gel so nutritious and nourishing? That is because apart from vitamins C and E, it also has a number of minerals, vitamin B12, and it made up of 88.3% water. That means it can be assimilated easily into your system after it has been digested, thanks to the water content. Is there any difference between a sweet gel or a bitter gel? This reminds me of a story I learned as a child. An ailing person went to one of the Wise men of the village, and asked for a medicine for one of his ailments. According to him, the previous medicine was not very effective, because it was not bitter. According to this patient, if the medicine was not bitter, how could it have a remedial effect upon the body?

The wise man smiled and told his young daughter who helped in the making up of medicines to add some magic leaves to the medicine. She immediately went into the garden, and picked up a handful of really bitter green leaves of the Neem. She added them to the medicinal tonic, and handed it over to the patient. The patient immediately applied a bit to a finger, licked it, and went home rejoicing. He had got the right medicine. This type of patient is very much present today, all over the World.

So if he finds himself confronted with a bitter piece of Aloe Vera, he is going to say hurrah, he can now eat this medicine as a sort of penance! But why make a face, when you are taking a little bit of Aloe Vera gel, all you need to do is start watering it more!

Aloe Vera takes a while to digest, after you have ingested it. That is the reason why I told you to drink a glass full of lukewarm water an hour after you have taken Aloe Vera juice, to help in the digestive process. Forget about those one liter bottles, unless you intend to use one bottle throughout your lifetime. Naturally, the best Aloe Vera is the one you have harvested fresh. That bottled stuff with all its preservatives is almost as bad as drinking juice concentrates made up of flavors, when you have fresh juice ready at hand.

Aloe Vera is an excellent diuretic. So if you find yourself suffering from any sort of liver or kidney ailments, try taking a little Aloe Vera gel, first thing in the morning, on an empty stomach. That is when it is going to benefit your system properly. One hour later, you are going to drink lukewarm water, and then eat your breakfast.

I saw a person recommended one tablespoonful of Aloe Vera juice, in which a pinch of turmeric- 3 grams - has been added to get rid of the kidney stones. He was given this medicine, first thing in the morning and then at night, before breakfast and after dinner. And he definitely does not have any kidney stones. No doubt, they dissolved due to the action of the turmeric and the juice and were removed from his body by his normal alimentary elimination processes.

An aunt of mine had a huge plant growing on her kitchen windowsill. She said that this was the best remedy for any sort of kitchen associated accidents, taking place while chopping, dicing, or cooking her huge meals. The moment she got a nick or a cut, she immediately rubbed fresh Aloe Vera gel, from the leaf onto that wound. Also, the moment anybody suffered from any sort of burn, fresh Aloe Vera gel was rubbed immediately on the affected areas so that there was no chance of the skin blistering or getting infected.

The dried bitter latex/sap which is normally found at the base of the Aloe Vera leaves is also known as "bitter aloes" in English. In medicine form, this powdered resin has been used in the Middle East and in Asia under the name of Aeluwah.

As I have already told you, drinking this juice in large quantities is going to have an adverse effect upon your health. Also, expectant mothers should not take Aloe Vera in any form, juice, gel, or bitter latex aloe powder internally either as a juice or a gel. That is because in ancient times, especially in Asia, Africa, and in the Middle East, this was given to mothers who did not want another child, so that they could miscarry naturally. And nursing mothers definitely did not drink or eat Aloe Vera.

Also, if you are trying Aloe Vera as a remedy for curing any disease, you are not going to eat any spicy foods or rich foods or sugars during this interval. If you are taking this as a general health enhancing tonic, you can take your daily diet in small quantities, and that may consist of occasional rich meals. Well, you are healthy, so you can afford to splurge a little on the meals of your choice, spicy, rich, and followed up with delicious sweet dishes.

Some More Aloe Vera Tips

Many have asked me whether it is necessary for you to get rid of the outer leafy portion, before you eat a piece of aloe leaf, and I've told them that traditionally, people who were so used to eating this, just used to snap off a piece, while walking past the plant, wash it, and pop it in their mouths. In the same way, they cut small pieces of the leaf, wrapped it in a piece of cloth, crushed it, and then squeezed the juice right into a bowl.

If you have the time and then the energy to boil the leaf, you can do that, and that means you have boiled gel to eat. The same boiled leaf can be put in a piece of cloth, crushed, and the juice extracted for future use.

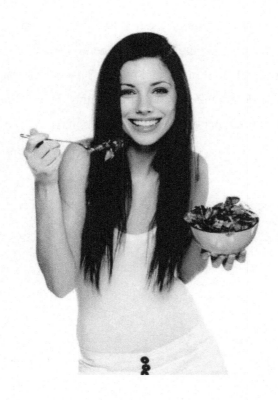

You can use the flowers of Aloe Vera as a delicious salad ingredient. They are edible and sweet smelling. Make up a mixture of cucumbers, spinach, mint, tomatoes, cabbage, and a little bit of other salad greens, and sprinkle with Aloe Vera flowers, finally topped with salad dressing, you have a tasty, healthy salad, ready at hand. You can add salt, lemons, pepper, and other herbs and spices to this mixture. If you want, you can also add olive oil.

So this is the traditional way in which you use an Aloe Vera leaf. Cut it, not completely from the stem, but half way, and allow it to still stay attached to the plant. Allow it to remain on the stem, uncut, for the next 10 minutes. The sap is going to flow out, and this is also very precious as latex. The leaf should be at least two years old. Now cut the leaf off completely, put on your gloves, and cut the spines.

Make a shallow cut, right through the middle of the leaf, exposing the gel inside. You can also remove the juice from the underside of the leaves. Scoop out the gel, and cut it into small pieces. This is now ready for consumption. You do not take more than 20 grams – one tablespoon full is 12.5 grams – of this gel, per day, and you always have to take it on an empty stomach.

Aloe Vera for Mouth Diseases

My friend, Astrid, told me about four years ago that she was using pure Aloe Vera gel as toothpaste, instead of the commercial toothpaste available in the market. Of course I laughed. But that lady is now in her 60s, does not suffer from any dental problems, gingivitis, bleeding of the gums, and swelling. This is because this gel is a perfect antiseptic.

Also, if you are suffering from any sort of mouth infection, as well as cold sores which are normally caused through viruses, the application of this gel on that affected area is going to yield very positive results. So I asked a dentist friend why she did not use this fresh gel as a natural healer, for patients suffering from root canal treatments, to heal the wounds naturally and without any sort of infection, she said that they did not like the bitter taste. But think of this as the best lubricant, antiseptic gel, and natural healer to get rid of any possible tooth infection or wound in the gums.

Here is another good use for Aloe Vera, especially in the removal of plaque. Just take some gel and rub it all over your teeth and gum area. This is going to remove the plaque buildup. It is also going to whiten the teeth, though how it does the whitening, I do not know– logical explanation is the plaque covering has gone, and the teeth have been exposed in all their natural beauty and splendor– and also, it prevents halitosis.

The gel toothpaste removes all the food particles sticking between your teeth, after you have eaten a meal. Also, if you have some teeth which are shaking loose on possibly diseased gums, just rub a little bit of gel all over that affected area. This is going to stop the pain, strengthen the gums, and if you do a little bit of supporting, by chewing up a few Aloe Vera gel pieces, this is going to give more power to your gums and teeth, literally and figuratively.

Astrid's Aloe Vera Gel Toothpaste

Remove the gel from inside a leaf, after the sap has been removed. Scoop it out, and put it in a glass jar, with a mouth just large enough into which you could put the head of your toothbrush. Now add just a pinch of salt to this gel, and use this morning and night, instead of your regular toothpaste to keep your mouth healthy.

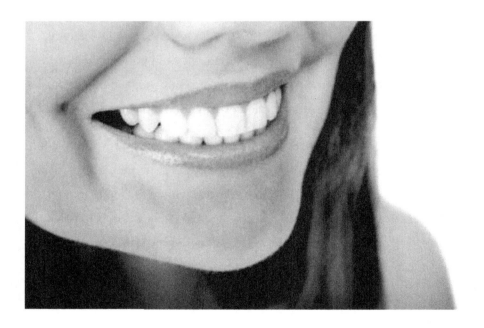

I found this toothpaste really good, especially when I knew that all the products were natural. But after that, I told her, Astrid, this needs stabilizing. She said, well, D, I make it in such small quantities that it does not get the chance to go bad, especially as her husband and her son also use this toothpaste.

So I told her that when she was going half of the way, to remove all that gel, and adding salt to it, for a healer and a whitener, she could stabilize it with a little bit of wheat germ oil. As I wanted to make sure that I did not suffer from any sort of dental problems, including gingivitis and halitosis, I was adding a teaspoonful of pure mustard oil, into the gel as a stabilizer and as a healing supporting ingredient –which as nearly every Easterner, brought up on Eastern, natural and ancient remedies– is the most powerful and healing combination available to man, when mixed with powdered salt.

This reminds me of one of the shaggy dog barmy Army tales, told to me by my grandfather, when I was a child – I do not know whether they were true, or he just made them up, as he went along. It was the Second World War. He was serving in Burma, under a British Colonel. Most of their soldiers were commando trained. Then he was a desk pusher, who had not been through any combat, during the whole of the war arrived on the scene, just to criticize and carp and cavil.

"How come the soldiers– especially the native ones – were not using toothpaste like Kolynos to clean their teeth?"

"That was because toothpaste had a distinctive smell, and any toothpaste foam, or soap foam, could give the enemy trackers the whiff and sign that there were enemy soldiers around. Because they had just had a soapy bath and brushed their teeth."

This was explained in a very patient tone, a bit reminiscent of *even a specimen like you should know that!*

But this desk pusher could not go against elementary hygiene, until the officer said that all the soldiers used salt to clean their teeth. Sometime later, Col. T. visited grandfather, in his native town, just as a friendly visit. And then he told grandfather, "It is lucky that your toothpaste made of salt did not have any mustard oil added to it, because I can smell it a mile off! Phew! This combination would have all of us cleaned out to a man."

When you use mustard oil, salt, plus Aloe Vera gel, it is not going to smell, when you rinse out your mouth with warm water, after the tooth cleaning is done.

So make your own gel toothpaste, right now and save on toothpaste and dental bills.

Heart and Chest Diseases

If you seem to be prone to respiratory, as well as chest infections, and you have an Aloe Vera plant around, you do not have to worry at all.

I am going to give you the traditional remedies for curing chest diseases. For this particular remedy, you need clarified butter. This is concentrated pure butter in a very powerful form, and has long been used in ancient times, to make up medicines.

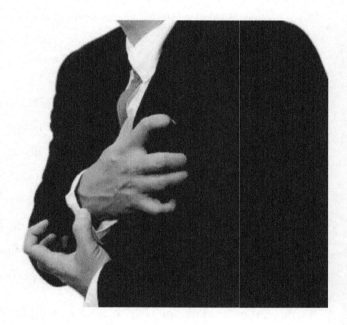

Take one teaspoonful of clarified butter. Just add a 2 inch piece of fresh Aloe Vera gel to this butter, and roast it on a griddle, slowly until the gel is pleasantly warm. Lick up the butter and gel combination with a spoon. This is the best remedy for a cough, which does not go away. You are going to take this three times a day on the first day, and also on the second day if necessary. By the second and third day, you are going to find yourself completely healed.

This is also excellent for a chronic old cold, or chest congestion, which does not appear to be healing naturally, Morning, afternoon, and night, roast your gel in clarified butter.

In the same manner, I was just trying out a natural remedy to cure a persistent wet cough. It appeared day before yesterday because I had neglected to wrap myself up well, before going out in the cold beginning of winter breeze. When I came back, there was this runny nose, and I knew that I was going to come down with a congested nose, chronic cough, and a muzzy head.

I just went into the garden, plucked off a leaf from the Aloe Vera plant, scooped out a piece of the gel, squeezed it until I could get one tablespoonful of fresh juice, added a little bit of honey, turmeric, and rock salt to this mixture, shut my eyes and gulped it down. Within three hours, I was bright eyed and bushy tailed, sniffing clearly all over the place and without any vestiges of a cough or a cold. Just one dose. If you allowed the cough to take hold, you would have to have at least three doses throughout the day. But, by the next morning, you would be perfectly all right.

Of course, it means that you have to wrap up your head and your feet, to prevent this problem from recurring again.

I saw someone making this traditional asthma and respiratory problem medicine, the traditional way. He took one kilo of fresh gel, put it in a piece of cloth after crushing it, and filtered it, until he had the juice. This juice was then put on slow heat, until the juice was reduced to half its original quantity. After that, he added 36 grams of rock salt to this gel and kept stirring it with a wooden spoon. When all the liquid content had evaporated, it was removed and the solid product powdered and placed in a glass bottle.

This is a very powerful medicine, so you are just going to take 250 milligrams. That is $1/14^{th}$ of a teaspoonful, with a teaspoonful of honey, once a day.

This is the best way in which you can get rid of a chronic chest infection, or asthma. Continue this until you are completely healed. It might take anywhere between 20 days to one month or more, depending on how severe your infection is.

When I asked him if he could make it in a clay utensil, he said yes, that could be done, but then he would be burning this in a clay oven. This method is just for reference, or for anybody who has a clay oven, the time, the energy, and the willpower to make a traditional method to cure any sort of chest infection permanently.

You take 250 grams of Aloe Vera gel. To this, you add 35 grams of rock salt. Now, put it in a clay pot, cover it, and seal the mouth with mud. Traditionally, this was cooked in a Potter's oven, for about the amount of the time it took for the Potter's utensils to be fired. The juice is reduced to a black powder. This medicine is so powerful that you just take one gram of this powder with raisins or rock candy. This is going to keep for years in a glass bottle, and you have enough of it to cure the chest infections of the whole town.

But, you say, you really do not have the time to allow this much juice to turn into ashes. So I am giving you my favorite shortcut, and other recipes, which just need you to take out one and a half teaspoons full of Aloe Vera juice, 1/6th teaspoon full of freshly ground pepper, 1/6th teaspoon full of ginger powder, and one tablespoon full of honey. Mix this up. You are going to take this mixture throughout the day, once in the morning and once in the evening. One and a half teaspoons full of Aloe Vera juice throughout the day is much more than enough!

You can also heat up the gel, on a griddle, take out the juice, add a little bit of honey and a little bit of clove powder to it, and lick the spoon. This is going to cure a persistent cough.

Heart Related Diseases

Now let us come to heart related diseases. Here also, you are going to see the wonders of Aloe Vera in action. Also, if you are suffering from high blood pressure, try this remedy.

Take 25 grams of fresh Aloe Vera juice, to which you have mixed six grams of rock candy and half a teaspoonful of roasted cumin powder. Take this mixture freshly made, morning and evening. This large quantity of Aloe Vera – 25+25 grams is needed to help cure your blood pressure, palpitations of the heart, and mild discomfort in the heart area.

If you are suffering from any pain in the heart region, you are going to do a little bit of massage, with this gel. As the skin is an organ which absorbs healing herbs and also heat, you are going to take two grams of powdered alum. To this, you are going to add some fresh Aloe Vera juice. Add a pinch of turmeric to this mixture. Make the patient lie down. Apply this paste all over the heart region, after roasting it well on the griddle.

Now take a warm cloth, and do some heating fomentation upon this paste. This is going to take away the pain slowly, as the heat gets absorbed in the heart region. If you do not have a cloth which can be warmed on the griddle, before applying the heated cotton on that paste, just take a hot water bottle in which you have put in hot water at a temperature which is not boiling, but is just right for fomentation.

When the patient is fast asleep after a sigh of relief – depends on how painful that heart pain was – you can put the bottle away for another day.

Aloe Vera for Stomach Ailments

Here is one particular recipe, which you might find very unusual, especially when you are cooking Aloe Vera. But in ancient times, it was cooked very often, and fed to the family, especially in the summers, where there was a chance of a summer epidemic affecting the area.

Take 200 grams of Aloe Vera gel. You are going to use pure clarified butter for cooking, because this is a food which is going to heal any pain in the stomach, which has been brought about through stomach ulcers, or any other infections. Take a tablespoonful of clarified butter. Put the chopped Aloe Vera gel pieces into the butter, and then add some cumin seeds.

This herb is excellent for healing purposes. Fry it gently and slowly on slow heat. Now add rock salt, rock candy, pepper, and a pinch of turmeric for seasoning and taste, according to whether you want it salty or sweet.

Hernia And Hydrocele

Hiatus Hernia

Normal

Sliding hiatus hernia

Paraesophageal hiatus hernia

This remedy was taught to me by my aunt, who used it on my granduncle, her father. He suffered from a hernia. So the moment it appeared she took two inches of Aloe Vera, and asked him to eat it. During this she took some Aloe Vera juice, added a little bit of rock salt to it, as well as a little bit of turmeric. She heated this mixture, spread it all over a piece of cotton cloth, and applied the cloth all over the affected hernia area.

This subcutaneous assimilation of Aloe Vera cured the hernia.

A hydrocele is a swelling in a testis. It normally occurs in newborn baby boys and goes away naturally. But many people do not know about it, and that is why doctors and quacks take plenty of advantage of this ignorance.

Sometime in 1999, our gardener came to my grandmother, looking really worried. He wanted her to lend him $50, which he could not afford. This was the amount being demanded by a doctor, who said that he was suffering from a hydrocele, it was a really serious condition, and he did not know anything about it, but he was worried about it, having lasting permanent harmful effects on his future childbearing capacities.

I happened to be there, and told him that the doctor had terrified him into a condition of panic stricken fear. Government health aid clinics treated this particular ailment as a routine, and all he had to do was to go to the government clinic, get an outdoor patient ticket made for $0.10, and he would be able to see a doctor who would operate on him free of cost.

He got the operation done that very weekend at the cost of $0.10. And he went around telling all the gardeners in the neighborhood that I had helped him so much, that occasionally I was asked what the cost of some particular operation should be, as demanded of them by the doctor and the right amount based on my knowledge of governmental medical programs. Within three months, all the doctors in the city got to know about me and wished that they could lay their hands upon me to commit justified wholesale pesticide.

If you do not have a free hydrocele treatment clinic in the vicinity, do not despair. Just take some fresh gel, add rock salt and turmeric to it and apply it to the affected area, twice a day in paste form. Wash it off, when you are taking your shower. This is going to be cured within a week.

Cirrhosis of the Liver and Enlarged Spleen

Cirrhosis of the liver normally occurs when a person is an alcoholic. And an enlarged spleen can occur due to an infection in the spleen area.

For cirrhosis, you need to cut up a leaf in small pieces. Boil it in water without peeling; remove the juice, sap, or gel. Remove the leaf, crush it, and filter it. The juice, 30 – 40 milliliters, has to be drunk, morning and evening, twice a day.

You can also add a little bit of black salt and ginger to this juice, to get rid of swelling in the liver and swelling in the spleen. It will take 10 days to cure you.

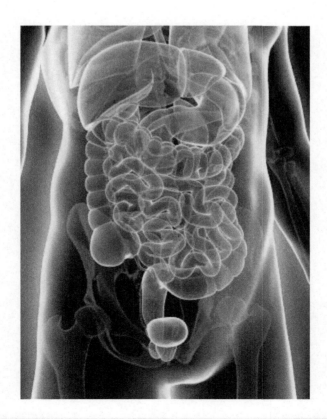

If you are worried about swelling in the spleen, you are going to make this traditional medicine and allow it to cook in the sun for one month. Take Aloe Vera juice, made up in water, as much as you'd like, and to this, you are going to add equal quantities of honey. So that means 20 tablespoons full of Aloe Vera juice and 20 tablespoons full of honey.

Put it in a glass bottle, and place it in the shade to cook for a month, in one corner of your balcony. After a month, you are just going to take five grams of this very powerful medicine after lunch and dinner, twice a day. You are going to mix it in a glass full of water first. Any sort of infection in your spleen is going to be healed, and any swelling is going to disappear. You take this juice, 15 minutes after you have had your lunch and dinner.

Dropsy And Hemorrhoids

In the same manner, if you know anybody suffering from dropsy, you could just tell him to start eating about one 1 inch piece of aloe gel every day.

Also, you can take one teaspoonful of Aloe Vera juice, three times a day. At night, the juice is going to take the form of one tablespoonful of juice to which you have added a little bit of dried ginger powder and pepper. This is going to cure the dropsy.

People suffering from fissures and piles were treated with fresh gel applied to that particular area, so that the fissures could be healed. People suffering from hemorrhoids should take in more fiber as well as more fresh fruit juice to heal the body naturally.

Doctors in Persia normally took out the gel, applied it on top of the bleeding hemorrhoid, and if they could manage to bandage it, bandaged it for half an hour. Let me tell you something amusing of ancient showmanship. This recipe called for the powdered skin of a snake added to this remedy. This of course was an exotic ingredient just added to impress the patient. The healing was done by the Aloe Vera gel.

Fissures were cured by applying a mixture of fresh gel mixed up with a little bit of castor oil, and bandaged. This helped heal the infection.

Even if you do not have stomach ailments, just eat a little bit of aloe gel every day. If you had any tendency to get hemorrhoids or piles, that would be cured internally. Also, any liver and kidney infections and enlargement of the spleen would be cured. But then, never overdo anything. If you eat too much aloe gel, you are going to suffer from swelling in the intestines, cramps, and blood passing in the stools.

This is a side effect, which a number of people all over the World are suffering, by eating Aloe Vera in large quantities, and by drinking large glasses of Aloe Vera juice!

People suffering from painful hemorrhoids can be cured within 15 to 20 days with just one leaf of Aloe Vera. Cut one leaf of Aloe Vera, fresh in the morning. Put it over a glass bottle and allow the sap to drip into the bottle. Now you are going to add 20 grams of the fresh Aloe Vera gel, right over the sap. Add just one gram of turmeric powder and 20 grams of powdered rock candy to this mixture.

You are going to get a powerful gel mixture. Feed it to the patient, 20 grams of rock candy is equal to one and a half tablespoons. You can feed it to him early in the morning, and then the rest of it to him at night.

It is going to take 10 days for your body to begin healing itself, and by the 20th day, you are not going to have any sort of hemorrhoid, painful piles, or even fissures. Also, if your body is all weak and pale, due to possible bleeding of your internal tissues, all this is going to be rejuvenated and healed with that Aloe Vera gel, and the Aloe Vera sap. The wet/dried sap is very powerful, and is dark yellow in color. Dried out, it is a powder, which is very much in demand by herbalists. Do not waste it ever.

Aloe Vera Bread

I was once fed bread made up of Aloe Vera juice! It contained 250 grams of freshly ground wheat flour, with the bran content still present, one tablespoonful of clarified butter, and one tablespoonful of Aloe Vera juice added to the mixture to make dough. To this dough were added pinches of rock salt, Bishops weed, just a pinch of roasted asafetida, pepper, and ginger powder. When the dough was ready for baking on a griddle, the cook rolled out a really thick piece of bread, flat with a rolling pin, like one would do a pastry or a taco or Pita.

After that, he heated up the griddle, applied some clarified butter on the surface, placed the bread on it, took a huge sack sewing needle and began to punch holes into the bread so that the butter could get absorbed in the cooking bread! The bread was then flipped over, in less than half a minute so that the under portion would not overcook.

And then I had to finish it with some homemade pickles, fresh butter, and buttermilk. I enjoyed the unusual combination, and thought, why not, a little bit of Aloe Vera gel, in a diet cooked could be a pleasant change.

According to the cook, he had learned this bread combination from his mother's grandmother! And she was a renowned cook, and never ever suffered from any sort of stomach problems, possibly brought up by eating many of her own rich and spicy dishes.

Conclusion

This book has given you plenty of information on how you can keep healthy with Aloe Vera. Aloe Vera is excellent as a preventative tonic. It is also a natural healer.

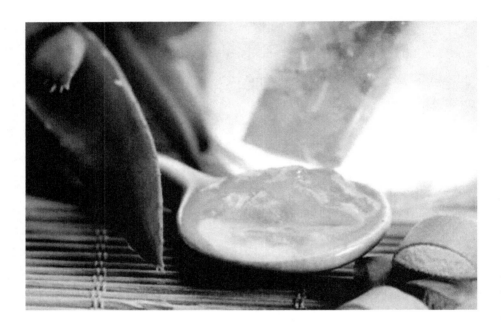

If you are feeling lethargic and rundown, and absolutely do not want to do anything, try this pick me up tonic. Take 30 grams of fresh Aloe Vera juice to which you have added 15 grams of pure honey and half a tablespoonful of lemon juice. Drink this morning and evening, and find your system perking up with this healthy natural tonic. Just take a spoonful of the gel, once a day and you are never going to suffer from any blood related problems, spleen, liver, or kidney problems ever.

I made up a mixture of ginger powder, rock salt, pepper – according to taste – and bishops weed, put it in the gel collected from three Aloe Vera leaves, and placed it in the sun – shade to dry. Within a week, I had a dried mixture, which I am still testing out to see, especially the problems it cures.

Digestive problem, a pinch of this mixture in warm water, twice a day, all ailments disappeared. Never suffered from a large spleen or cirrhosis of the liver, but the liver is functioning properly and well. I do not take more than three grams at a time.

So, one really can consider Aloe Vera to be a cure all, as the ancients knew well.

Live Long and Prosper!

Author Bio

Dueep Jyot Singh is a Management and IT Professional who managed to gather Postgraduate qualifications in Management and English and Degrees in Science, French and Education while pursuing different enjoyable career options like being an hospital administrator, IT,SEO and HRD Database Manager/ trainer, movie , radio and TV scriptwriter, theatre artiste and public speaker, lecturer in French, Marketing and Advertising, ex-Editor of Hearts On Fire (now known as Solstice) Books Missouri USA, advice columnist and cartoonist, publisher and Aviation School trainer, ex-moderator on Medico.in, banker, student councilor ,travelogue writer … among other things!

One fine morning, she decided that she had enough of killing herself by Degrees and went back to her first love -- writing. It's more enjoyable! She already has 48 published academic and 14 fiction- in- different- genre books under her belt.

When she is not designing websites or making Graphic design illustrations for clients , she is browsing through old bookshops hunting for treasures, of which she has an enviable collection – including R.L. Stevenson, O.Henry, Dornford Yates, Maurice Walsh, De Maupassant, Victor Hugo, Sapper, C.N. Williamson, "Bartimeus" and the crown of her collection- Dickens "The Old Curiosity Shop," and "Martin Chuzzlewit" and so on… Just call her "Renaissance Woman" - collecting herbal remedies, acting like Universal Helping Hand/Agony Aunt, or escaping to her dear mountains for a bit of exploring, collecting herbs and plants, and trekking.

Check out some of the other JD-Biz Publishing books

Gardening Series on Amazon

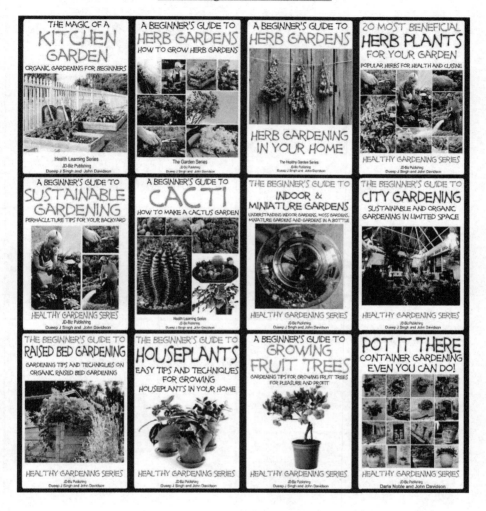

Download Free Books!

http://MendonCottageBooks.com

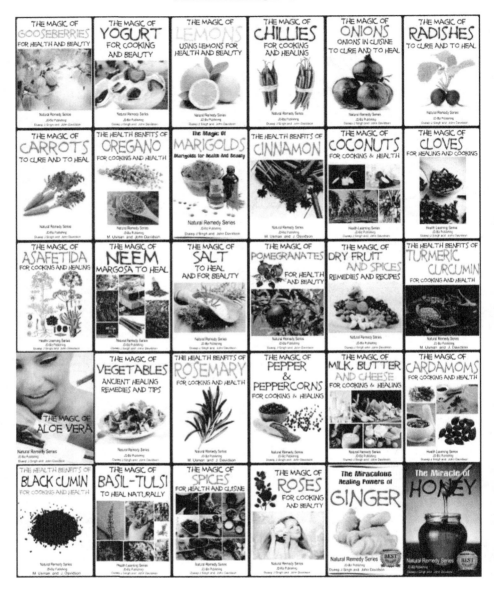

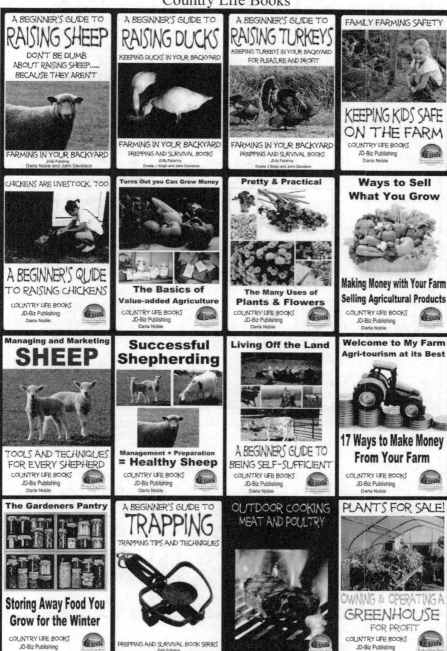

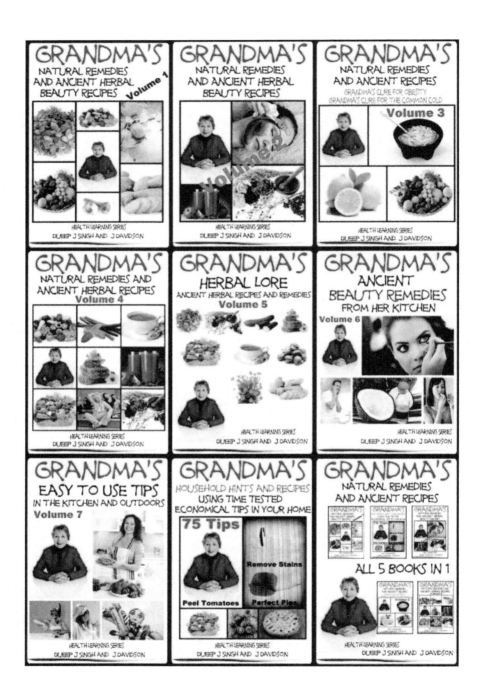

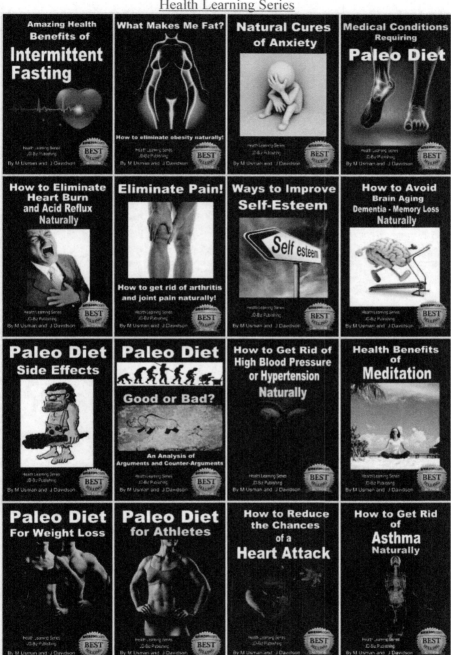

Amazing Animal Book Series

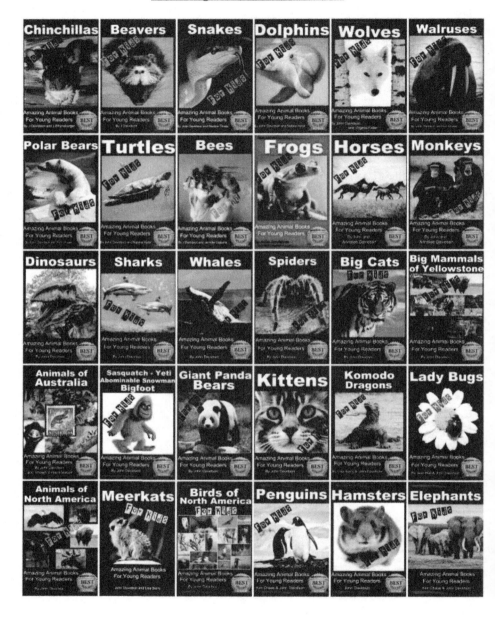

Learn To Draw Series

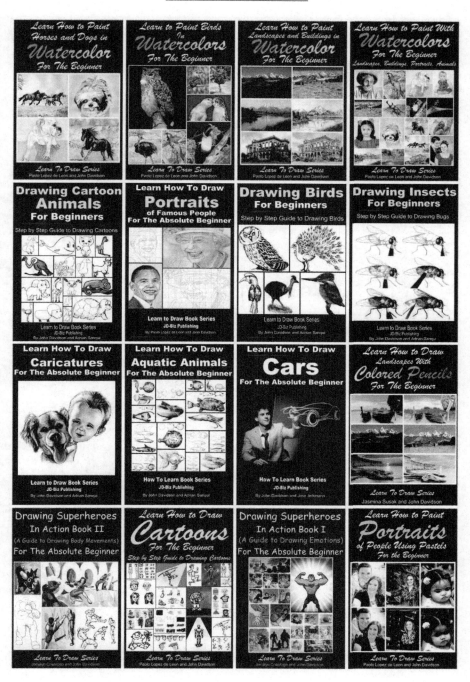

How to Build and Plan Books

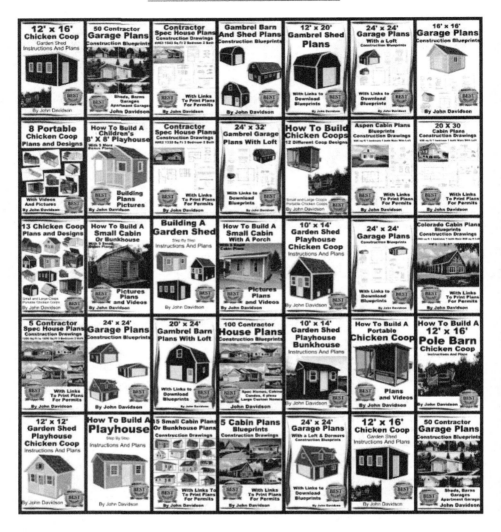

Entrepreneur Book Series

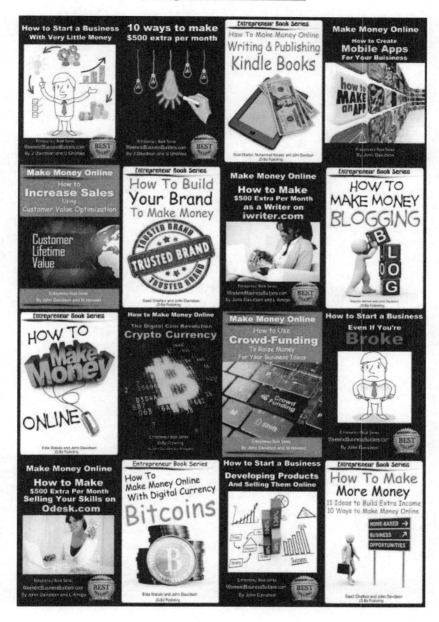

Our books are available at

1. Amazon.com

2. Barnes and Noble

3. Itunes

4. Kobo

5. Smashwords

6. Google Play Books

Download Free Books!

http://MendonCottageBooks.com

Publisher

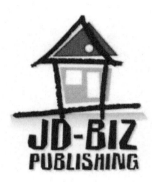

JD-Biz Corp

P O Box 374

Mendon, Utah 84325

http://www.jd-biz.com/

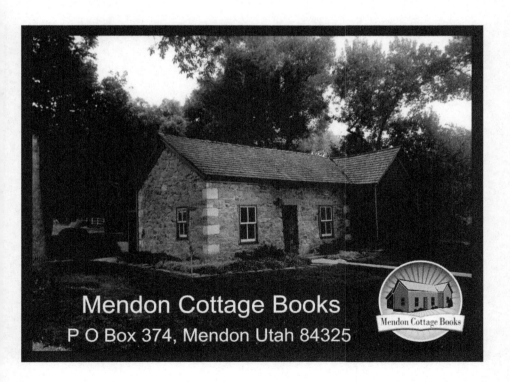

Mendon Cottage Books

P O Box 374, Mendon Utah 84325

Printed in Great Britain
by Amazon

42925473R00030